Fibromyalgia

Understanding, managing, and improving Fibromyalgia and its signs and symptoms!

Table Of Contents

Introduction

I want to thank you and congratulate you for downloading the book, "Fibromyalgia".

This book contains helpful information about Fibromyalgia, what it is, and how to treat and improve it.

You will learn about the different signs and symptoms of Fibromyalgia, along with the potential causes of this condition. This book also explains how Fibromyalgia is diagnosed by a medical professional.

Included are the most common medical treatments for Fibromyalgia that your doctor may prescribe you. There are also alternative therapies, and self-help strategies provided that will assist the medical treatments in managing Fibromyalgia.

This book will provide you the steps and strategies required to successfully manage and improve your Fibromyalgia once and all for all. Fibromyalgia can be a difficult diagnosis to live with. However, with the help of the strategies provided in this book, it's possible to live a healthy, successful, and fulfilling life, even with Fibromyalgia present!

Thanks again for downloading this book, I hope you enjoy it!

Chapter 1:
Understanding Fibromyalgia

Fibromyalgia (FM) is a combination of the Latin word "fibro", which means fibrous tissues and the Greek words "myo" and "algia", which stand for muscle and pain, respectively. Literally, it means pain of the connective tissues and muscles. The name exactly describes the medical condition, as unexplained widespread pain in muscles and joints is the primary symptom of FM. It is also referred to as fibromyalgia syndrome (FMS) as there are other presenting symptoms associated with it.

A Brief History

For centuries, FM was oftentimes mistaken as a form of mental disorder. Health experts back then thought that the patients were making up the complaints of pain, and that these were simply formed by their imagination. This is not surprising as pain is highly subjective and relative. In addition, there is currently no specific diagnostic or laboratory test to determine the presence of pain.

With complaints of aches, tiredness, difficulty sleeping and stiffness, FM was initially called "muscular rheumatism". In the early 1900's the medical name was changed to "fibrositis", attributing inflammation as the cause of pain. In 1976, fibrositis was changed to fibromyalgia, as inflammation was no longer considered as the culprit of the pain. In 1981, a scientific study finally confirmed the presence of symptoms of pain and tender points in the body. This paved the way for FM to be finally accepted and understood as a medical condition.

Some Statistics on FM

FM is a non-threatening chronic condition affecting one out of 50 people in the US alone, reaching an estimate of 4 to 5 million Americans afflicted with it. Hence, it ranked second as the most common ailment involving the musculoskeletal system, with osteoarthritis as first. It affects women more than men with a ratio of 7:1. Studies show that 60% of the diagnosed patients are in their 30-40's while 35% are either in their 20's or between 50-60's. The percentage of children being affected by this condition is around 5%.

Causes of FM

The exact cause of FM remains unknown, however, several factors are considered as probable causes of this medical condition.

- ➢ Genetics. FM is noted to have familial tendencies, meaning there is an increased likelihood of developing the disease if a member of the family is diagnosed with it. The specific gene has not yet been named though.

- ➢ Other medical conditions. Some diseases tend to trigger the development of FM. Most of them are rheumatic conditions, meaning the affected areas are the bones, joints or muscles. Examples of these are:

  - o Lupus – a multi-organ autoimmune disease that affects joints, kidneys, heart, lungs, skin, blood cells and the brain.

  - o Osteoarthritis – pain, stiffness and swelling of joints.

- o Ankylosing spondylitis – an inflammatory disease affecting the spine.

    - o Rheumatoid arthritis – an inflammatory disorder of the joints.

    - o Temporomandibular disorder (TMD) – pain in the jaw, jaw joint and surrounding facial muscles.

- ➢ Chemical imbalances in the central nervous system (CNS). Low levels of serotonin, dopamine and noradrenaline in the brain are said to contribute to the development of FM. With the imbalances in these substances, disruption in the system that pertains to pain occurs. This leads to patients becoming extremely sensitive to pain and pressure. Regulations of sleep, mood, appetite, response to stress, and behavior are also affected.

- ➢ Stress. Exposure to stressful events has been reported to trigger or aggravate FM. Both physical and mental traumas can make a person more prone to FM.

Although FM is not fatal, it can cause serious physical, mental, emotional, social, and even spiritual distress to the afflicted. However, one can still enjoy a normal and happy life even if he or she is diagnosed with Fibromyalgia. Understanding the disease and knowing what to do are the keys to ensure that FM will not take control of a person's life.

Chapter 2:
Recognizing The Symptoms of Fibromyalgia

The initial complaint of the person with FM is widespread pain that lasts for three months or more. Pain is considered widespread when there is an occurrence of it on both sides of the body, plus below and above the waist. Its pain is oftentimes described as a constant dull ache. Aside from muscle and joint pains, spasms and tightness can also be experienced, intensifying the pain.

There is also allodynia. This is a feeling of heightened pain to things that normally should not cause pain. An example of allodynia includes experiencing excruciating pain when light touch and slight pressure is applied. Allodynia is a prominent symptom of people with fibromyalgia. Ischemia or failure to deliver oxygenated blood to certain parts of the body is considered as the main cause. When the body part is deprived of oxygen, even for a very short time, it creates an environment for inflammation. The actual sensitivity pain comes from the phenomenon when the body is trying to re-infuse oxygen to these oxygen-deprived parts. Stronger free radicals are released. Examples are superoxide, peroxynitrite and nitric oxide. This is called "reperfusion injury".

Fibromyalgia is also called Fibromyalgia syndrome because there are other symptoms that go with it other than widespread pain and allodynia. Here are some of them.

1. Persistent and chronic fatigue. Even after several hours of sleep, people with FM wake up feeling tired. The fatigue is described as flu-like. This can be attributed to sleep disorders associated with FM. Though the person

may be able to sleep during bedtime, it would be very light and not refreshing. Pain also keeps them awake sometimes. Feelings of tiredness are experienced even with minimal exertion.

There is also a lack of energy, enthusiasm and motivation, causing the person to be withdrawn to other people, happenings and other forms of socialization. Eventually, this affects his or her relationships with other people, be it in the workplace, school, community, or family.

A lack of appetite further contributes to the lack of energy of the patient. Serotonin, one of the neurotransmitters being affected by FM, is responsible for regulating appetite. A poor appetite results in decreased levels of serotonin. The body has no source of energy when the patient is not eating due to lack of appetite.

2. Sleep difficulties. Sleep disturbances are caused by several factors. First, pain prevents the person from achieving a restful sleep. This becomes a cycle, as lack of sleep, on the other hand, would exacerbate pain. Since the pain is widespread, there is no comfortable position that the person can assume to facilitate a good sleep. Hence, the patient is kept awake trying to position himself or herself comfortably.

Second, the disturbance in the chemical balance is also being pointed out as a culprit in causing irregular sleep patterns. Serotonin is the one that regulates sleep. The disruptions in the hormones affect neurotransmitters, which in turn will cause the message (regarding sleep) being relayed to the brain to be delayed or to be not delivered at all.

3. Stiffness. As many as 90% of FM patients suffer from stiffness, especially in the morning after being in bed for several hours. It usually lasts 30 minutes to 1 hour before the patient can move normally. The stiffness can persist the whole day but at a lesser intensity. The exact reason for the stiffness remains a mystery to health authorities. One probable cause is the natural instinct of a person to avoid movement of a painful part. Thus, there is decreased blood flow to it, aggravating the pain. Another probable cause is again the effect of an imbalance of chemicals in the brain. Lack of exercise is also a possible factor.

4. Digestive disorders. This may include bloating, diarrhea, constipation or a combination of these three. Around 70% of FM patients experience this symptom. This may occur due to increased sensitivity of the patient to pain, which stimulates stomach upsets, leading to digestive disorders. Another possibility is that it is the side effect of prescribed drugs for FM, especially NSAID's (non-steroidal anti-inflammatory drugs).

5. Fibro or Brain fog. A cognitive difficulty that hinders the ability of the person to focus or pay attention to mental tasks. There is also confusion, memory lapses, and word mix-ups. The popular theories concerning this symptom are due to lack of sleep, and depression. Poor perfusion or delivery of oxygenated blood to the brain is also cited as a possible reason. Recent studies are pointing to chronic pain as the culprit of brain fog.

6. Headaches and migraines. Around 70% of FM patients complain of severe headaches and migraines. The probable cause is the presence of myofascial trigger points (knots in the shoulder and neck muscles).

7. Depression. Serotonin is called the happiness hormone, as it is the one responsible for regulating moods and preventing depression. In patients with FM, this hormone is disrupted. In turn, patients feel irritated and depressed. Another hormone, dopamine, is also affected by FM. A lack of dopamine can lead to a lack of enthusiasm, feeling of bad moods, and an inability to concentrate.

8. Imbalance. Risk of falls and accidents is common with FM patients. One reason is imbalance. Studies have led the researchers to measure the leg strength of FM patients, and the results have shown that FM patients have lesser leg strength. The following factors were considered for this: poor delivery of oxygenated blood to the legs (as these body parts are far from the heart already), and a lack of sleep.

9. Itchy skin. The majority of FM patients also suffer from itching or burning skin. Early studies have pointed out the presence of immune-reactive proteins in high concentration found just beneath the skin. The body perceives these proteins as foreign objects, causing the body to release histamine and cytokines, which in turn cause the itchiness or burning feeling of the skin.

These symptoms are chronic. They sometimes come and go. There are also factors that can cause flare-ups of FM symptoms. It would be best for FM patients to avoid the following factors when possible to prevent experiencing the symptoms. These are:

 ➢ Change in weather, especially cold climate.

 ➢ Hormonal fluctuations. For instance before a menstrual period or during menopausal stage

 ➢ Stress

 ➢ Lack of sleep

 ➢ Anxiety

 ➢ Depression

 ➢ Loud noises

 ➢ Strong odors

 ➢ Bright lights

 ➢ Prescription medicines

 ➢ Some foods

These factors, in turn, could cause the following symptoms:

 a. Chest pain that is not related to any heart disorder

 b. Difficulty in breathing

 c. Dizziness

 d. Palpitations

 e. Numbness and tingling sensations

f. Profuse sweating

g. Dry or burning eyes and mouth

h. Painful periods

FM is a chronic disease and you can expect the symptoms to disappear and then be back again after several months. Treatment is needed to manage the symptoms and to allow the person to assume a normal life and schedule. In the proceeding chapters, you'll find out how fibromyalgia is diagnosed, and learn the different ways to manage and control the signs and symptoms of FM.

Chapter 3:
Laboratory and Diagnostic Examinations For Fibromyalgia

Fibromyalgia is oftentimes misdiagnosed. Most probably because the presenting symptoms are general and may be present in other medical conditions too, such as arthritis, chronic fatigue syndrome, depression and lupus. Also, the symptoms are highly subjective, meaning the doctors would depend on the patient's description and feelings to identify the disorder. This is quite tricky as each person has a unique tolerance and threshold for pain.

Most of the time, the doctors order different lab tests, not to diagnose FM alone, but to rule out the other possible medical disorders. As a result, it may take several months or even years before a correct diagnosis is made. A delayed diagnosis is equivalent to delayed treatment, which in turn, will cause more discomfort for the patients.

In reality, laboratory examinations will not actually help in diagnosing FM. These tests are ordered not to confirm FM, but to assess the presence of other medical conditions. This is because FM always yields normal lab results. If the doctor suspects that you have a medical condition that might co-exist with FM, he or she may order the following exams:

Complete blood count – this checks the red blood cell count (RBC). A decreased production of RBC leads to anemia, which is one probable reason for fatigue. It also assesses the count of white blood cells (WBC). An increased WBC count is indicative of the body's response to foreign substances invading the body.

ESR or erythrocyte sedimentation rate – is also a blood test used to identify the presence of inflammation. Lupus, for instance, will yield a positive result for ESR.

C-reactive protein (CRP) – just like ESR, it also checks for inflammatory responses in the body.

ANA or antinuclear antibodies test – this is a specific blood test to ascertain the diagnosis of lupus.

Thyroid hormone test – this test checks thyroid gland activities. It may result in a hyperactive, normal or hypoactive gland activity.

Blood calcium – Calcium plays a role in muscle contraction. Low levels of calcium in the blood can cause muscular cramps.

Kidney and liver tests – this is to ascertain if there are damages to these organs. It could also serve as baseline data prior to the prescription of medicines.

Cholesterol level – the doctor may also want to determine if the cholesterol level is within a normal range. When tissue perfusion is compromised already, a high level of cholesterol might aggravate the situation as it can cause blockages in the arteries, further causing poor delivery of oxygenated blood.

Rheumatoid factor – Normally, the body produces antibodies to fight and eliminate invading viruses, bacteria and other harmful microorganisms to protect the body. Rheumatoid factor antibody can cause undetected damage to the body because they attach to normal body tissue without any reactions from the body. 50-80% of patients with rheumatoid arthritis will have positive results of this test.

X-Rays – this is used to determine the extent of damage to the bones as caused by arthritis. X-Rays will yield normal results when checking for the tender points of fibromyalgia.

When the following exams are taken and the results have ruled out other medical diseases, a diagnosis of FM will be made on these three criteria:

1. There is widespread pain all over the four quadrants of the body.

2. The pain is present for 3 months or more.

3. The patient is negative for other diseases.

The doctor will also evaluate the patient's trigger points, investigate about the causes of fatigue and sleep disturbances, evaluate the level of stress, and refer the patient to a psychologist or psychiatrist to test for depression. There are usually no diagnostic procedures being done to FM patients.

As soon as FM is confirmed, the doctor and the patient will plan a multifaceted treatment program that would be applicable to the patient. This may include medications, lifestyle modification, alternative therapies, and other self-care activities.

Chapter 4:
Pharmaceutical Management For Fibromyalgia

As there are many presenting symptoms of FM, there are also be many drugs that the doctor will prescribe to relieve the patients from their discomforts. These may include sleeping pills, antidepressants, and pain relievers. The goal of the therapy is to achieve a normal life for the FM patients.

Pharmaceutical management may differ from one patient to another, as each person will react uniquely to the therapy. Therefore, the doctors usually resort to a trial and error process in finding the perfect pharmaceutical regimen that will be ideal for a certain patient. Hence, reporting of the effectiveness of the drugs to the doctor is vital to ascertain the right regimen for the patient.

It was only recently that three drugs were FDA-approved to specifically treat fibromyalgia. These are Lyrica (pregabalin), Cymbalta (duloxetine hydrochloride), and Savella (milnacipran HCl). Lyrica is an anticonvulsant drug that is used to treat neuropathic pain and partial seizures. It has been found to treat generalized anxiety disorder, too. Cymbalta is a selective serotonin and norepinephrine reuptake inhibitor antidepressant (SSNRI). It balances the chemicals in the brain, thereby preventing depression. Savella is also an SSNRI.

In the treatment of FM, Savella is first used. As Savella allows more neurotransmitters in the body, that in turn would permit more neuron to neuron communication. This drug can amplify the effects of endorphins – also known as the body's natural painkillers. The effects would be a decrease in pain, less fatigue, and an overall feeling of wellbeing. Depression is also avoided with the use of Savella. The down side, however, are the side effects. Savella and other tricyclic antidepressants can cause dry eyes and mouth, dizziness, drowsiness and constipation, to name just a few.

Here are other drugs that may be prescribed to relieve the symptoms of FM.

Pain relievers. To help reduce the pain and improve sleep, the patient can take over the counter pain relievers like ibuprofen, acetaminophen and naproxen sodium. Prescription pain relievers include tramadol. To avoid stomach upsets and other complications such as nausea and vomiting, heartburn, bleeding, and stomach ulcers, these pain relievers are best taken with meals or when the patient is full. The frequency is every 4-6 hours only, or as prescribed by the doctor. The patient should not take painkillers for more than 10 days. As narcotics can cause dependence, these are not prescribed for FM patients unless the pain is too unbearable. Caution must be observed to avoid the development of addiction to these drugs.

Antidepressants. To ease the pain and fatigue, antidepressants such as Milnacipran (Savella), and Duloxetine (Cymbalta) are prescribed. To promote sleep, the doctor might order amitriptyline or fluoxetine.

Anti-seizure drugs. Some medicines for epileptics are found useful in the reduction of pain. This could be attributed to the relaxation of the muscles that these drugs cause. These are known as Gabapentin. The first drug to be FDA-approved, Lyrica, to be used for FM, falls under this category.

Compliance to pharmaceutical therapy is vital to ensure that FM patients are free from debilitating symptoms. These drugs aim to allow patients to live normal lives in spite of having Fibromyalgia.

Chapter 5:
Alternative or Complementary Therapies To Manage Fibromyalgia

In addition to pharmaceutical therapy and a healthy lifestyle (cessation from smoking and drinking alcoholic beverages, proper diet, exercise, rest and sleep), patients are often prescribed alternative and complementary therapies to combat FM. These therapies are designed to induce rest and sleep, relax muscles, manage stress, fight depression, and reduce pain for FM patients.

Here are some of the alternative/complementary therapies:

1. Acupuncture. This therapy helps in increasing blood flow to all parts of the body. When this occurs, pain decreases. Symptoms of brain fog, headaches and migraines can also be lessened. Aside from this, this therapy is known to increase the production of endorphins – the body's natural painkillers. Acupuncture is done through the insertion of thin needles into the skin. There is another method of acupuncture, called electro-acupuncture, which allows a minimal electric current to run through the needles. Both methods help relieve fibromyalgia. Acupuncture is reported to relieve FM patients of anxiety and fatigue.

2. Massage. Pain is relieved due to a reduction of muscle tension. As a massage is done to FM patients, circulation of blood is also improved. This causes the release of natural chemicals of the body which aid in the suppression of depression, irritability and mood swings. Plus, massage therapy promotes rest and sleep. A 20-minute massage a day is recommended. Swedish

massage, which focuses on the superficial layers of muscles, uses kneading, long strokes and friction techniques. Deep tissue massage, using elbows and thumbs, is also beneficial to release muscle tension.

3. Heat therapy. The application of moist heat can improve blood circulation and promote the relaxation of tensed muscles. One can also do simple heat therapy home-fixes like taking a warm shower, or warming clothes by putting them in the dryer before wearing them.

4. Chiropractic treatment. This is adjustment of the spine. The goal of the therapy is to increase the mobility of the spinal column through stretching, exercising, and massaging of the spine.

5. Meditation. Freeing the mind from worries and stresses allow it to be rested. This provides a calm and peaceful mood, which will benefit both the body and mind of the patient. In addition, it also provides nourishment to the spirit, creating hope and a more positive outlook toward life.

6. Progressive muscle relaxation. Stress can result in tensed muscles. A technique that will help eliminate this problem is progressive muscle relaxation. With this, the patient practices correct breathing patterns as he or she tenses and then relaxes each muscle from head to foot. This series of tension and relaxation of the muscles results in overall relaxation of the muscles.

Symptoms of FM can return or be aggravated because of feelings of depression. To fight off depression, here are some of the recommended actions to take:

➢ Cultivate supportive relationships. Depressed people have a tendency to withdraw and isolate themselves from others. However, to win the battle against depression, the support of significant others is very important. Therefore, both the patient and the family must work together to overcome depression. They may even undergo family therapy to have a better understanding and management of the disease. Support groups don't only include loved ones and family members. The patient's network of relationships can extend to the members of the health team, friends, coworkers, and even new acquaintances in support groups.

➢ Challenge negative thinking. Depressed people are often pessimistic. They feel hopeless most of the time and their thoughts are clouded with negative expectations. FM patients are empowered by challenging those negative thoughts and changing them into positive ones. This can be done through positive self-talk, affirmations from themselves and other people, and the intentional and forceful rejection of negative thoughts.

➢ Self-care management. The goal is for the patient not to be totally dependent on others. As the patient develops a desire to help himself or herself, depression is being overcome. Practicing healthy habits such as sleeping 8 hours a day, ceasing smoking and other unhealthy habits, exercising, eating right, and socializing with others, are things that one can do. However, this takes discipline and strong will, as there will be times when the patient won't feel like doing these things for themselves.

Combine pharmaceutical therapy with these alternative therapies and the symptoms of FM will be manageable. Life can and will go on, even if one has FM.

Chapter 6:
Life With Fibromyalgia

To be diagnosed with fibromyalgia is not an easy thing. However, don't think that this is the end of the road for you. People with fibromyalgia can enjoy a normal, successful, and happy life.

Gaining a thorough understanding of the illness is the first step to take. Aside from this book, look around for other information that will increase your knowledge about fibromyalgia. There are other avenues through which you can learn how to manage this medical condition such as a health team, support groups, books, and online data.

A positive attitude is also a key in having a successful life in spite of having fibromyalgia. When you focus on the positive things, like having your family, or being able to do numerous things like work or study, you strengthen yourself and allow life to go on, with or without FM. However, when all your energy and thoughts are on FM alone and its negative effects on your body and mind, you allow the disease to take control of your life.

As mentioned, modifying your lifestyle will help greatly. Here are some tips you can use to improve your lifestyle:

1. Sleep. Although people with FM find this very difficult to accomplish, here are some strategies that might work so that sleep can be obtained:

   a. Do not try to oversleep. Sleeping more than what your body requires could prove unhelpful to FM patients. Instead of trying to sleep as much as one can, try to curtail the sleeping time. This way, sleep is more solid rather than fragmented.

b. Keep a sleep diary. Doing this may reveal some data as to why you can sleep at certain times, but struggle to at others. Use this information to combat sleep pattern disturbances.

c. Practice consistency. Having a regular time for sleeping and waking up will strengthen the circadian cycling.

d. Use relaxation techniques. There are many available techniques that one can use to ensure a relaxed state, which will lead to improved rest and sleep.

e. Avoid strenuous activities and heavy meals three hours before sleep. Doing this will keep your body in an excited state, making sleep more difficult to attain. Exercise is best done in the morning.

f. Shorten your daytime nap if you have one. This will allow for a longer sleeping time at night.

g. Make the bedroom a conducive place to rest. Take note and adjust the temperature, lighting, cleanliness, and sound that may interfere with sleep. Use the bedroom for sleeping purposes only. Do not watch television, read books or do your office work there. When the mind is set that the bedroom is exclusively for sleeping only, it will prepare the mind and body for sleep once you let yourself in the bedroom.

2. Exercise. The presence of stiffness and muscle pain causes FM patients to avoid exercise and other physical

activities. However, doing this will actually lead to more pain. Although it will be uncomfortable at first, exercising is a must as it is one of the keys to overcoming the symptoms of FM. Here are some tips to help you be successful with developing an exercise regime:

a. Know the importance of exercise. In treating fibromyalgia, exercising is beneficial as it can strengthen muscles and bones, reduce stress, improve balance, and maintain bone mass. Plus, it helps maintain an ideal weight, which is important for someone with FM.

b. Start slow. Don't jump straight in to heavy exercise is you currently live a sedentary lifestyle. Try to increase your everyday activities first before you start an exercise regimen. How? Lessen TV time or other activities that keep you seated or lying down for a long period of time. Instead, try to have more time doing something productive and active like simple gardening, walking the dog or taking a stroll in the park. When you are used to being active, start the regimen with brisk walking for five minutes at first, three times a week. Increase the time as you continue the regimen. This may seem slow at first but the goal is consistency rather than quantity.

c. Listen to your body. Although movement is encouraged, your body will also give you signs of how well it is coping with the increased physical activity. Look for signs and symptoms that suggest that you're overdoing it. Adjust the activities according to your body's response.

d. Be consistent. Do something everyday. You can do walking, cycling, yoga, or low impact exercises. If you can find an exercise buddy, that would be better. Use stairs instead of elevators or escalators. Every little thing counts.

e. Adjust your workout. As you progress in this area, try to add other activities that might help. Do this with the help and instruction of a professional trainer. It is also a standard procedure that you inform your doctor about your exercise regimen.

Note: The effects of exercises might not be so obvious at first and you might really find it hard to do this because of the pain. Be patient. This is a proven method to relieve one of FM symptoms. It might take 6 months or more before the benefits of exercise can be fully felt and enjoyed.

3. Diet. Studies are still being undertaken as we speak to link diet with the reduction or elimination of symptoms of FM. Although the studies are not yet conclusive, here is some information that you can use to your advantage in combatting FM symptoms:

a. Certain foods can trigger symptoms. What are these foods? Nobody can really specify as it varies from person to person. However, foods with additives seem to be the main culprit. Even without an official statement from health researchers, a lot of doctors are advising their FM patients to refrain from eating foods with additives. Stick to natural and organic foods. You can also determine if certain foods in your diet can trigger FM by keeping a food journal. Simply write down all your food intake for a day for one month or more (depends on you), and then under remarks, place any untoward incidents that occur to you. Check if the occurrence of incidents goes together with a certain food. Avoid that food for eight weeks. Afterwards, try to eat it again. If you experience the same reactions, then permanently avoid that food.

b. Eat foods rich in Vitamin D. A deficiency in this vitamin can be the cause of muscle and bone pains. It would also help if you expose yourself to early morning sunshine to augment your supply of Vitamin D. During wintertime, Vitamin D supplements could be helpful.

c. Consume more omega 3-fatty acids. These can be found in fish (salmon, tuna, herring and others), walnuts, and flaxseeds. They are said to be helpful in reducing inflammation and preventing cardiovascular diseases. Again, there are supplements that you can take to provide the needed omega-3 fatty acids.

d. Avoid coffee. As sleep disturbance is a major problem in patients with fibromyalgia, ditching the coffee will be beneficial. Some patients take coffee to make them more active in the morning, however, this could backfire at night.

e. Eat more fresh and green vegetables. These are rich in antioxidants. Remember, pain can be caused by the increased release of free radicals in the body. Antioxidants can curb these free radicals and reduce pain in the process.

When it comes to diet, it is not only about what and how much to eat, but when to eat as well. The recommended timing is small, frequent feeding.

Final words on fibromyalgia

Fibromyalgia can be controlled and managed. One can do things that make life enjoyable even when you are diagnosed with fibromyalgia. Today, take charge of your life. Be in control. Understand that a happy and successful life is attainable, even with fibromyalgia.

Conclusion

Thank you again for downloading this book!

I hope this book was able to help you learn more about Fibromyalgia!

The next step is to put this information to use, and begin managing and improving your own Fibromyalgia condition!

Finally, if you enjoyed this book, please take the time to share your thoughts and post a review on Amazon. It'd be greatly appreciated!

Thank you and good luck!